GAO

Report to the Subcommittee on Oversight of Government Management, the Federal Workforce, and the District of Columbia, Committee on Homeland Security and Governmental Affairs, United States Senate

July 2012

INFLUENZA PANDEMIC

I0426053

Agencies Report Progress in Plans to Protect Federal Workers but Oversight Could Be Improved

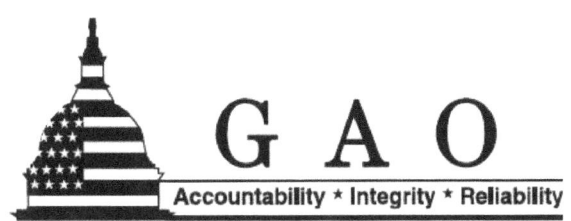

G A O
Accountability * Integrity * Reliability

GAO-12-748

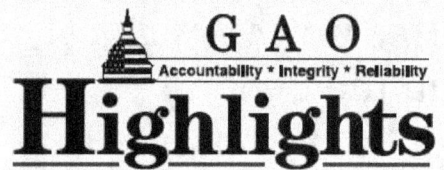

GAO
Accountability * Integrity * Reliability

Highlights

Highlights of GAO-12-748, a report to the Subcommittee on Oversight of Government Management, the Federal Workforce, and the District of Columbia, Committee on Homeland Security and Governmental Affairs, United States Senate

INFLUENZA PANDEMIC

Agencies Report Progress in Plans to Protect Federal Workers but Oversight Could be Improved

Why GAO Did This Study

Federal agencies must plan to protect federal workers essential to ensuring the continuity of the country's critical operations in the event of a pandemic. GAO reported in 2009 that agencies had made uneven progress in developing operational influenza pandemic plans and some agencies were not close to having plans. In addition, there was no real mechanism to monitor agencies' progress.

GAO was asked to (1) determine what progress federal agencies report they have made since GAO's 2009 report and identify challenges federal agencies report they face in protecting their workforce during an influenza pandemic, and (2) determine the extent to which oversight of agencies' progress is being conducted and how the oversight information is being used.

GAO surveyed the 24 agencies covered by the Chief Financial Officers Act of 1990, conducted a follow-up case study review, and interviewed agency officials responsible for providing guidance to other federal agencies in planning for an influenza pandemic.

What GAO Recommends

GAO recommends that DHS provide additional oversight of agencies' pandemic preparedness and help focus attention on areas of uneven progress reported in GAO's survey by directing FEMA to include in its biennial assessments of agencies' continuity capabilities consideration of agencies' progress in assessing exposure risk levels of occupational exposure, identifying appropriate protective measures, and establishing operational plans to provide such protections for federal workers during an influenza pandemic. DHS concurred with the recommendation.

View GAO-12-748. For more information, contact Stanley Czerwinski at (202) 512-9110 or czerwinskis@gao.gov

What GAO Found

In 2012, federal agencies reported they had made progress in planning to protect their federal employees during an influenza pandemic. For example:

- Twenty-three of 24 federal agencies reported they had completed influenza pandemic plans that address the operational approach they would use to protect their employees in the event of an influenza pandemic. In 2009, 20 agencies reported completing such plans.

- All 24 agencies reported that, to reduce employees' risk of exposure to influenza, they developed policies or procedures such as telework and avoiding all unnecessary travel. In the 2009 survey, 22 agencies reported developing the former policy and 18 the latter.

- All of the agencies reported that they planned for the distribution of hygiene supplies to protect employees whose duties require them to work onsite during an influenza pandemic. In 2009, 18 agencies reported taking this planning step.

However, the agencies reported uneven status in some key areas suggesting some additional oversight is needed. For example, only nine agencies reported they have classified all or most jobs for onsite mission essential functions by exposure risk level. Additional oversight could help in ensuring that, by classifying jobs by exposure risk level, agencies have appropriate measures in place to protect those employees who must carry out mission essential functions that cannot be performed remotely during an influenza pandemic.

There is limited oversight of agencies' progress to protect their employees during a pandemic. In 2008, the Homeland Security Council required agencies to certify their pandemic planning status, but according to agencies' officials, has not done so since then. As in 2009, GAO interviewed four agencies—Department of Health and Human Services, Department of Homeland Security (DHS), Department of Labor, and Office of Personnel Management. Each of these agencies is responsible for providing influenza pandemic continuity of operations guidance, which includes elements such as planning, personnel protection, or workplace options to federal departments and agencies. DHS and the Federal Emergency Management Agency (FEMA) reported they conduct biennial assessments of department and agency continuity capabilities and report the results to the President through the National Continuity Coordinator. However, this assessment does not include planning elements specific to influenza pandemic planning, such as whether federal workers' influenza pandemic risk assessments are regularly updated and whether agencies have planned to provide protective measures to mitigate exposure risks. Including such information in the biennial assessment process could provide monitoring, evaluation, and reporting of progress and help focus attention on those areas in which reported progress is uneven.

Contents

Letter		1
	Background	4
	Agencies Reported Progress in Planning to Protect Employees during an Influenza Pandemic	6
	Agencies' Plans and Progress to Protect Federal Workers During an Influenza Pandemic Receive Limited Oversight	29
	Conclusions	33
	Recommendation For Executive Action	34
	Agency Comments	34

Appendix I	Chief Financial Officers Act Agencies	36

Appendix II	List of Agencies and Selected Components	37

Appendix III	Objectives, Scope, and Methodology	38

Appendix IV	Comments from the Department of Homeland Security	40

Appendix V	GAO Contact and Staff Acknowledgments	42

Related GAO Products		43

Table		
	Table 1: List of Agencies with Selected Components	15

Figures		
	Figure 1: Agencies Reported Progress in Completing Influenza Pandemic Plans	7

Figure 2: All Agencies Reported Plans to Protect Federal Workers through Use of Social Distancing Strategies and Hygiene Supplies   9
Figure 3: Agencies Reported Progress Employing Additional Protective Strategies   10
Figure 4: All Agencies Reported Progress in Making Human Capital Information Available to Employees   11
Figure 5: Agencies Reported Testing Various Information Technology and Telecommunications Capabilities   12
Figure 6: Majority of Agencies Reported Requiring Components to Complete Influenza Pandemic Plans   14
Figure 7: Selected Components' Influenza Pandemic Planning Efforts   16
Figure 8: Agencies Reported Using Various Social Distancing Strategies to Avoid Situations that Increase Workers' Risk of Exposure for Selected Components   17
Figure 9: Selected Components' Facility-Level Influenza Pandemic Plans   18
Figure 10: Use of Various Social Distancing Strategies in Facility-Level Influenza Pandemic Plans   19
Figure 11: Agencies Reported Identification of Onsite Mission Essential Functions and Determination and Notification of Employees Tasked With Such Functions   20
Figure 12: Agencies Reported Uneven Status in Classifying Jobs by Exposure Risk Level for Onsite Mission Essential Functions   22
Figure 13: Many Agencies Reported Classifying Jobs by Exposure Risk Level for Selected Component's Onsite Mission Essential Functions   23
Figure 14: Most Frequently Reported Challenges in Planning for Federal Worker Protection for an Influenza Pandemic   24

Abbreviations

ATO	Air Traffic Organization
CDC	Centers for Disease Control and Prevention
CFO Act	Chief Financial Officers Act of 1990
Commerce	Department of Commerce
COOP	continuity of operations
DHS	Department of Homeland Security

DOD	Department of Defense
DOE	Department of Energy
DOT	Department of Transportation
Education	Department of Education
EPA	Environmental Protection Agency
evaluation tool	*Continuity Evaluation Tool*
FAA	Federal Aviation Administration
FEMA	Federal Emergency Management Agency
GSA	General Services Administration
HHS	Department of Health and Human Services
HSC	Homeland Security Council
HUD	Department of Housing and Urban Development
Implementation Plan	*National Strategy for Pandemic Influenza Implementation Plan*
IT	information technology
Key Elements	*Key Elements of Departmental Pandemic Influenza Operational Plans*
Labor	Department of Labor
NASA	National Aeronautics and Space Administration
NCC	National Continuity Coordinator
NOAA	National Oceanic and Atmospheric Administration
NRC	Nuclear Regulatory Commission
NRF	*National Response Framework*
NRR	Office of Nuclear Reactor Regulation
NSC	National Security Council
NSF	National Science Foundation
NSS	National Security Staff
OPM	Office of Personnel Management
OSHA	Occupational Safety and Health Administration
SARS	Severe Acute Respiratory Syndrome
SBA	Small Business Administration
SSA	Social Security Administration
State	Department of State
Treasury	Department of the Treasury
USAID	U.S. Agency for International Development
USDA	Department of Agriculture
VA	Department of Veterans Affairs

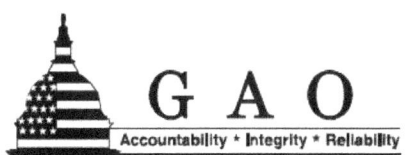

July 25, 2012

The Honorable Daniel K. Akaka
Chairman
The Honorable Ron Johnson
Ranking Member
Subcommittee on Oversight of Government Management, the Federal
Workforce, and the
    District of Columbia
Committee on Homeland Security and Governmental Affairs
United States Senate

During an influenza pandemic many federal employees will be able to
perform their agencies'[1] mission essential functions[2] remotely through
telework arrangements, but other federal employees, such as air traffic
controllers, will have to work at assigned locations where there will be an
increased chance of infection due to proximity to others. Anxiety and
concern over working during an influenza pandemic could reduce the
number of critical federal employees available to work. For example,
researchers who studied the attitudes of emergency pre-hospital medical
care providers concluded that absenteeism could significantly impair the
community's frontline medical response.[3] Among the reported lessons
learned from the 2003 outbreak of Severe Acute Respiratory Syndrome
(SARS) in Toronto was that although health care workers have a duty to

---

[1]Throughout this report, we use "agencies" to refer to all parts of cabinet-level
departments (e.g., Department of Transportation) or independent agencies (e.g.,
Environmental Protection Agency), including headquarters-level components, operational
components, and field-based entities.

[2]According to the Department of Homeland Security's Federal Continuity Directive 1,
mission essential functions are described as the limited set of agency-level government
functions that must be continued throughout, or resumed rapidly after, a disruption of
normal activities. Mission essential functions are those functions that enable an
organization to provide vital services, exercise civil authority, maintain the safety of the
general public, and sustain the industrial and economic base during disruption of normal
operations.

[3]C. Irvin, L. Cindrich, W. Patterson, and A. Southall, "Survey of Hospital Healthcare
Personnel Response during a Potential Avian Influenza: Will They Come to Work?"
Prehospital and Disaster Medicine, vol. 23, no.4 (2008): 328-335. F. Archer, M. Coory, K.
Jamrozik, H. Kelly, S. Raven, V. Tippett, and K. Watt, "Anticipated Behaviors of
Emergency Prehospital Medical Care Providers during an Influenza Pandemic."
Prehospital and Disaster Medicine, vol. 25, no.1 (2010): 20-25.

provide care, institutions have a reciprocal duty to support health care workers so they can do their jobs as effectively and safely as possible.[4]

The Homeland Security Council's (HSC)[5] 2006 *National Strategy for Pandemic Influenza Implementation Plan* (Implementation Plan)[6] required federal agencies to develop operational influenza pandemic plans that provide for the health and safety of their employees and ensure the agency will be able to maintain its essential functions and services in the face of significant and sustained absenteeism. According to the Implementation Plan, an operational influenza pandemic plan should articulate the manner in which the department, including its components,[7] plans to discharge its responsibilities to support the federal efforts in fighting an influenza pandemic; address the operational approach to employee safety and continuity of operations; and describe how the department plans to communicate with its stakeholders. The challenges that agencies must address include (1) identification of onsite mission essential functions that must be continued and those employees who must perform them and (2) implementation of workforce strategies and measures to protect those employees who must continue such functions. We reported in 2009 that agencies' progress was uneven in influenza pandemic planning and some agencies were not close to having operational influenza pandemic plans.[8] We also reported that the Federal

---

[4]S. Benatar, M. Bernstein, A. Daar, B. Dickens, S. MacRae, R. Shaul, P. Singer, R. Upshur, and L. Wright, "Ethics and SARS: lessons from Toronto." *BMJ*, vol. 327 (2003): 1342-1344.

[5]The HSC was established pursuant to Executive Order 13228, on October 8, 2001, for purposes of advising and assisting the President with respect to all aspects of homeland security and serving as a mechanism for ensuring (1) coordination of homeland security-related activities of executive departments and agencies and (2) effective development and implementation of homeland security policies. Congress subsequently established the HSC for the purpose of more effectively coordinating the policies and functions of the federal government relating to homeland security. See Homeland Security Act of 2002, Pub. L. No. 107-296 (Nov. 25, 2002), 6 U.S.C. § 491 and § 494.

[6]HSC, *National Strategy for Pandemic Influenza Implementation Plan* (Washington, D.C.: May 2006).

[7]Components refer to subordinate entities of departments such as component agencies, field or regional offices, or other operating divisions. For example, the Federal Aviation Administration is a component of the Department of Transportation.

[8]GAO, *Influenza Pandemic: Increased Agency Accountability Could Help Protect Federal Employees Serving the Public in the Event of a Pandemic*, GAO-09-404 (Washington, D.C.: June 12, 2009).

Aviation Administration (FAA) faced unique challenges protecting air traffic controllers who must perform essential onsite functions during an influenza pandemic.

In June 2009, we reported that there was no mechanism in place to monitor and report on agencies' progress in developing influenza pandemic plans to protect their workforce and recommended that the HSC request that the Department of Homeland Security (DHS) monitor and report to the Executive Office of the President on the readiness of agencies to continue their operations while protecting their employees in the event of a pandemic. The HSC noted that it would give serious consideration to our report findings and recommendations, and DHS said the report findings and recommendations would contribute to its efforts to ensure that government entities are well prepared for what may come next. Given the importance of agencies' ability to continue operations while protecting their employees in the event of an influenza pandemic, you asked us to (1) determine what progress federal agencies report they have made since our 2009 report and identify challenges federal agencies report they face in protecting their workforce during an influenza pandemic; and (2) determine the extent to which oversight of agencies' progress was being conducted and how the oversight information is being used.

To address these objectives, we surveyed the 24 agencies covered by the Chief Financial Officers Act of 1990 (CFO Act) to determine whether they made progress in their preparedness to protect their workforce since our 2009 survey and to identify challenges they faced in planning for protection of their workers. All 24 CFO Act agencies completed the survey for a response rate of 100 percent. In addition, to better understand the extent to which influenza pandemic planning had filtered down to the component and facility levels, we also gathered data from these levels in our 2012 survey. In our 2009 survey, 15 of 24 agencies provided examples of key component-level mission essential functions that could not be performed remotely during an influenza pandemic. Using those examples, we selected a component from each of these 15 agencies for our 2012 survey and surveyed the agencies to determine whether they had made plans at lower organizational levels to protect their employees whose onsite presence was necessary in order to carry out mission essential functions. In addition to these surveys, we conducted follow-up work to assess FAA's progress in addressing the unique challenges we highlighted in our 2009 report regarding protection for air traffic controllers who must perform onsite mission essential functions during an influenza pandemic. Further, we analyzed documentation of oversight activities and interviewed officials from the Department of Health and Human Services (HHS), DHS, Federal Emergency Management Agency (FEMA), Department of Labor's (Labor) Occupational Safety and Health Administration (OSHA), and the Office of Personnel Management (OPM), who were tasked with providing guidance, policy, or influenza pandemic related expertise to other federal agencies in planning for an influenza pandemic. Lastly, we reviewed the Implementation Plan, *National Response Framework* (NRF),[9] our prior work assessing influenza, and other relevant literature to help inform our analyses.

We conducted this performance audit from July 2011 through July 2012 in accordance with generally accepted government auditing standards. Those standards require that we plan and perform the audit to obtain sufficient, appropriate evidence to provide a reasonable basis for our findings and conclusions based on our audit objectives. We believe that the evidence obtained provides a reasonable basis for our findings and conclusions based on our audit objectives. Detailed information on our scope and methodology appears in appendix III.

Background

The federal government employed over 4.3 million federal employees throughout the United States and abroad in 2010.[10] Federal employees perform functions across a multitude of sectors, from those vital to the long-term well-being of the country—such as environmental protection, intelligence, social work, and financial services—to those directly charged with aspects of public safety—including corrections, airport and aviation safety, medical services, border protection, and agricultural safety.

In the event of any emergency, federal employees responsible for their agencies' mission essential functions will be expected to continue them in order to sustain agency operations. Unlike incidents that are discretely bounded in space or time (e.g., most natural or man-made disasters), an influenza pandemic is not a singular event, but is likely to come in waves, each lasting weeks or months, and pass through communities of all sizes

---

[9]DHS, *National Response Framework* (Washington, D.C.: January 2008).

[10]OPM, "Historical Federal Workforce Tables: Total Government Employment Since 1962," accessed July 17, 2012, http://www.opm.gov/feddata/HistoricalTables/TotalGovernmentSince1962.asp.

across the nation and the world simultaneously, as we have witnessed with the 2009 H1N1 influenza pandemic. While a pandemic will not directly damage physical infrastructure such as power lines or computer systems, it threatens the operation of critical systems by potentially removing the essential personnel needed to operate them from the workplace for weeks or months because of illness, the need to care for family members who are sick, or fear of becoming infected.

In response to concerns that the emergence of H5N1 avian influenza (or bird flu) in Asia in 2003 would mutate and result in a human influenza pandemic, the President and his HSC issued two planning documents. Issued in November 2005, the *National Strategy for Pandemic Influenza*[11] provides a high-level overview of the approach that the federal government will take to prepare for and respond to an influenza pandemic. The Implementation Plan issued in May 2006 lays out the broad implementation requirements and responsibilities among the appropriate federal agencies, including that agencies have operational influenza pandemic plans that address the protection of federal employees, and clearly defines expectations of nonfederal entities.

To help federal agencies plan for and respond to an influenza pandemic, the HSC issued the *Key Elements of Departmental Pandemic Influenza Operational Plans* (Key Elements),[12] a checklist for federal agencies to use in planning their influenza pandemic preparedness. The checklist includes elements covering plans and procedures, essential functions and services, safety and health for their employees, communications, human capital, and information technology (IT) capabilities. The Key Elements also reference Federal Continuity Directives 1 and 2, which guide the identification of mission essential functions,[13] and instructs agencies to include functions that cannot be deferred for 12 weeks or more without

---

[11]HSC, *National Strategy for Pandemic Influenza* (Washington, D.C.: November 2005).

[12]HSC, *Key Elements of Departmental Pandemic Influenza Operational Plans* (Washington, D.C.: August 2008).

[13]In February 2008, the Secretary of Homeland Security released two federal continuity directives: Federal Continuity Directive 1 provides direction for the development of continuity plans and programs for the federal executive branch, and Federal Continuity Directive 2 provides additional guidance for agencies in identifying their mission essential functions.

impact to an agency's mission and nonessential functions that can be suspended temporarily during an influenza pandemic.

We reported in June 2009 that the HSC requested that federal agencies certify to the council that they were addressing applicable elements of the Key Elements checklist in December 2006 and October 2008.[14] Because the certification process, as implemented, did not provide for monitoring and reporting as envisioned in the Implementation Plan, we recommended in our June 2009 report that the HSC request that the Secretary of Homeland Security monitor and report to the Executive Office of the President on the readiness of agencies to continue their operations while protecting their employees in the event of an influenza pandemic. In commenting on our report, the Acting Executive Secretary of the HSC noted that the report made useful points regarding opportunities for enhanced monitoring and reporting within the executive branch concerning agencies' progress in developing plans to protect their workforce. The official also noted that the council would give serious and careful consideration to the report findings and recommendations. We will discuss HSC and DHS's efforts in more detail later in the report.

Agencies Reported Progress in Planning to Protect Employees during an Influenza Pandemic

---

[14]GAO-09-404.

Additional Agencies Reported Completing Influenza Pandemic Plans to Protect Their Federal Workers

As shown in figure 1, almost all of the agencies we surveyed—or an increase of three agencies since 2009—reported in 2012 that they have completed influenza pandemic plans[15] that address the operational approach for how they would protect their federal employees in the event of an influenza pandemic. HHS reported that while they will continue to work towards a final document, they recognize the need for continuous improvement and incorporation of lessons learned. They describe the draft influenza pandemic plan as a "living document" that allows for continuous updates. Because of that, they do not have a target date for when a final plan will be completed. Additionally, HHS is supporting a series of research studies on the effectiveness of respirators or surgical masks to prevent influenza infection and to better understand their role in workforce protection. HHS reports that pandemic planning is an ongoing process that is shaped by lessons learned in the field as well as improvements in the medical and scientific research base.

Figure 1: Agencies Reported Progress in Completing Influenza Pandemic Plans

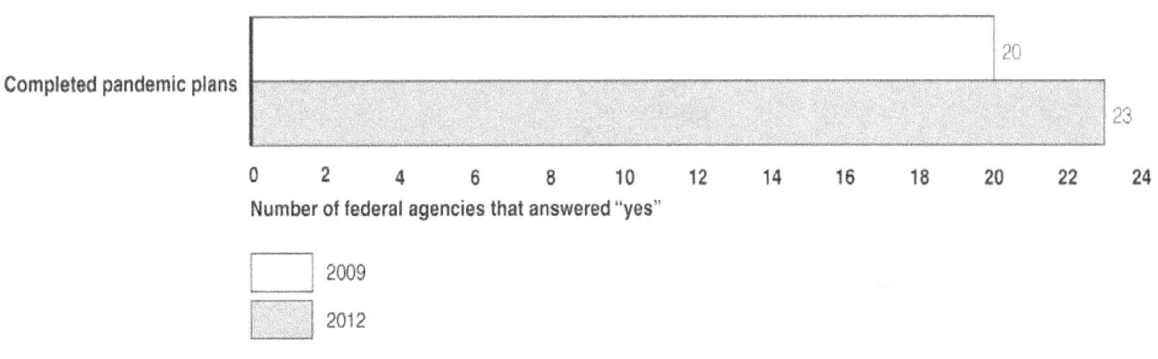

Source: GAO analysis of 2009 and 2012 agency survey responses.

In addition, 20 agencies reported that their influenza pandemic plans addressed how they would protect federal employees who maintained mission essential functions that could not be performed remotely during an influenza pandemic. Of the four remaining agencies, three of them—including the Department of Education (Education), General Services

---

[15]For purposes of our survey, we defined "pandemic plan" as any document that contained information related to an influenza pandemic. Specifically, a pandemic plan could be a standalone plan or part of a broader plan (e.g. annex to an all-hazards plan or continuity of operations (COOP) plan).

Administration (GSA), and Small Business Administration (SBA)—reported all of their mission essential functions could be performed remotely, and the U.S. Agency for International Development (USAID) reported that its plan was being updated to include this information.

Agencies Reported Progress Incorporating Protective Strategies into Their Influenza Pandemic Plans

According to OSHA guidance on protecting workers, the best strategy to reduce the risk of becoming infected with influenza during an influenza pandemic is to avoid crowded settings and other situations that increase the risk of exposure to someone who may be infected. If it is absolutely necessary to be in a crowded setting, the time spent in a crowd should be as short as possible. Some basic hygiene and social distancing[16] precautions, such as encouraging employees to wash their hands or use a hand sanitizer after they cough, sneeze, or blow their noses, can be implemented in every workplace.[17] Figure 2 shows progress agencies reported to have made incorporating various protective strategies since 2009. Specifically, all of the agencies reported that they developed policies or procedures consistent with this strategy such as telework and avoiding all unnecessary travel. They have also planned for the distribution of hygiene supplies to protect employees whose duties require their presence at an assigned workplace during an influenza pandemic.

[16]OSHA defines social distancing as reducing the frequency, proximity, and duration of contact between people to reduce the chances of spreading influenza pandemic from person-to-person.

[17]OSHA, *Guidance on Preparing Workplaces for an Influenza Pandemic*, OSHA 3327-02N 2007.

Figure 2: All Agencies Reported Plans to Protect Federal Workers through Use of Social Distancing Strategies and Hygiene Supplies

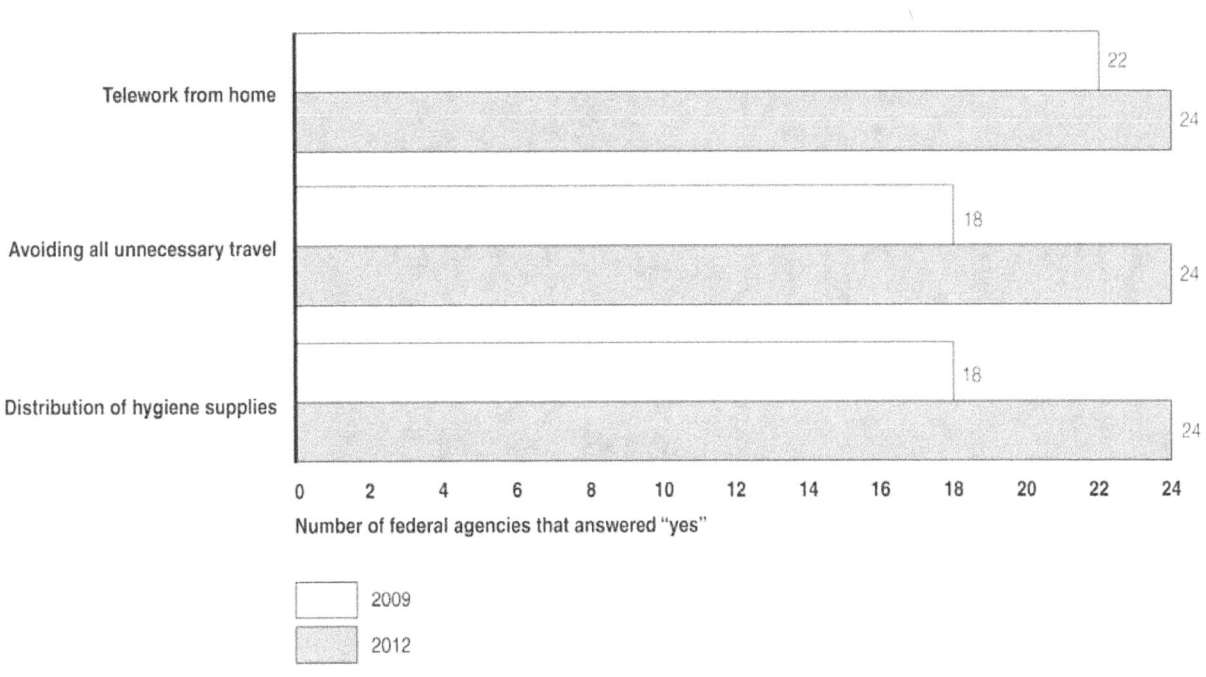

Number of federal agencies that answered "yes"

2009
2012

Source: GAO analysis of 2009 and 2012 agency survey responses.

Moreover, as shown in figure 3, agencies reported an increase over 2009 in a variety of other actions that could reduce the risk of exposure for federal workers, including the use of flexible schedules to reduce the number of employees who must be at work at one time or in one specific location and implementing pandemic influenza-specific office protocols such as no-handshake policies. However, not all of these actions may be applicable to all workplace settings.

Figure 3: Agencies Reported Progress Employing Additional Protective Strategies

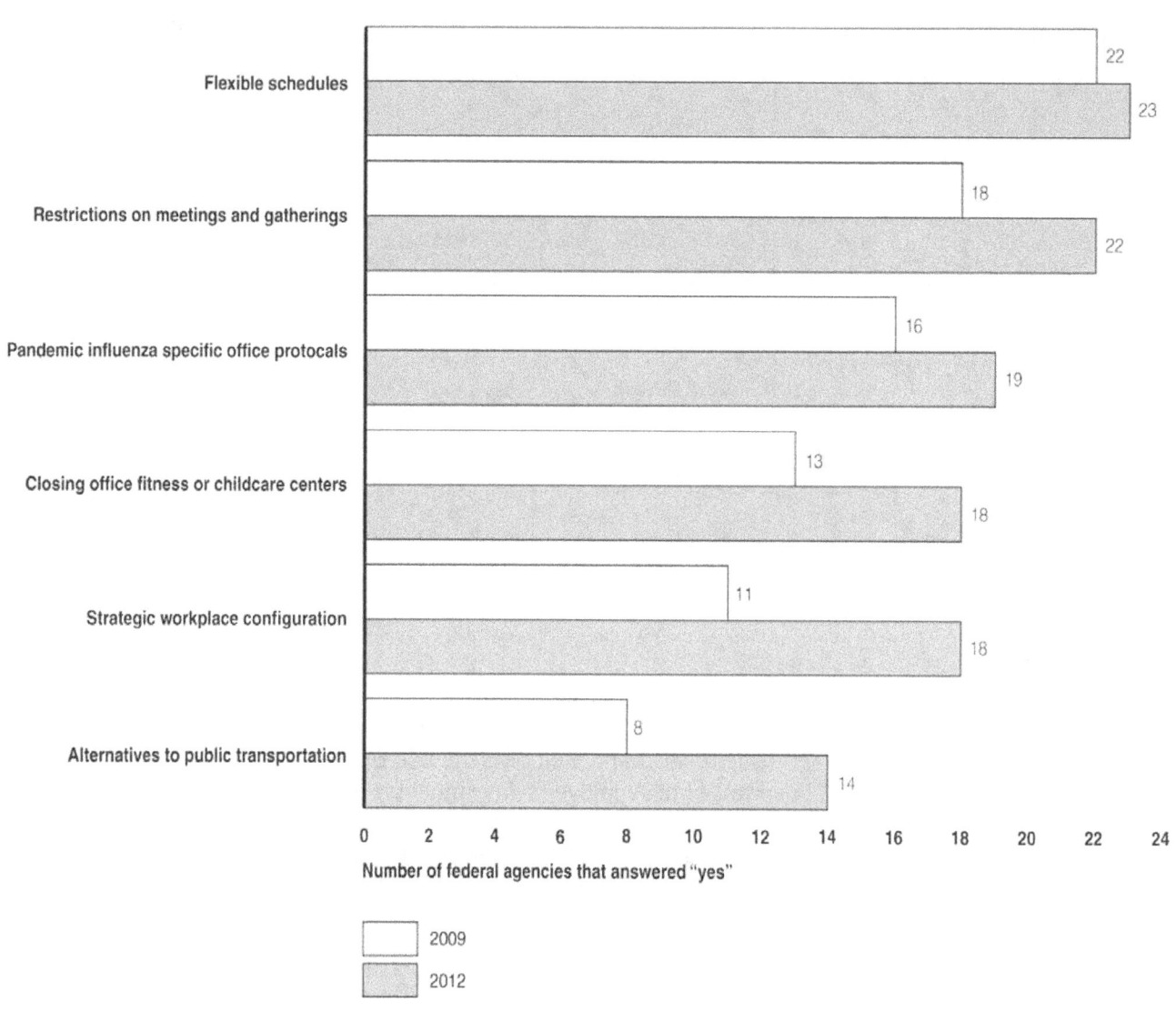

Number of federal agencies that answered "yes"

☐ 2009
▨ 2012

Source: GAO analysis of 2009 and 2012 agency survey responses.

GAO-12-748 Influenza Pandemic

All Surveyed Agencies Reported Providing Human Capital Information to Employees

According to Federal Continuity Directive 1, agencies must implement a process to communicate human capital guidance for emergencies, such as pay, leave, staffing, and other human resources flexibilities, to employees to ensure continuity of mission essential functions during an emergency. Given the potential severity of an influenza pandemic, it is important that employees understand the policies and requirements of their agencies and the alternatives, such as telework, that may be available to them.

While a majority of agencies surveyed in 2009 reported they had made information available to employees on how human capital policies and flexibilities would change in the event of an influenza pandemic, figure 4 shows that all surveyed agencies reported in 2012 that they have made such information available to their employees.

Figure 4: All Agencies Reported Progress in Making Human Capital Information Available to Employees

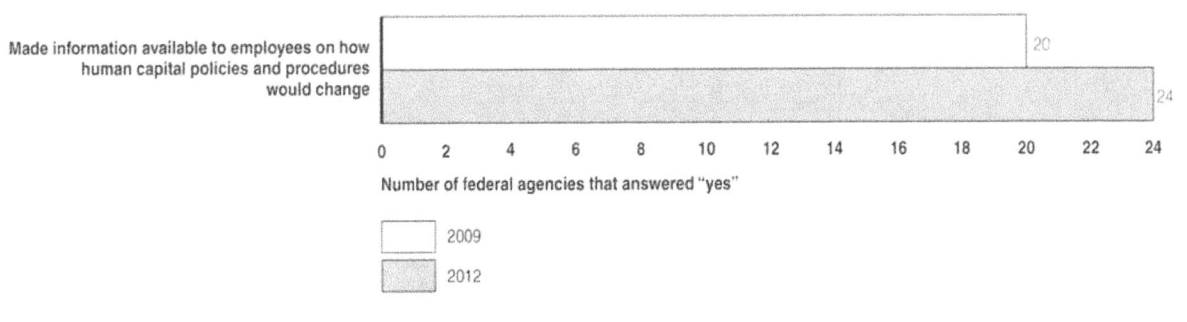

Source: GAO analysis of 2009 and 2012 agency survey responses.

Almost All Agencies Reported Testing IT Capabilities for Handling Telework during an Influenza Pandemic

As noted earlier, all of the agencies reported that they developed policies or procedures for using telework in the event of an influenza pandemic. In our 2012 survey, we asked agencies if they had tested the various modes of IT and telecommunications capabilities to ensure that they would be capable of handling employees working remotely during an influenza pandemic. As shown in figure 5, almost all of the agencies reported to have tested e-mail, teleconferencing, intranet access, and access to vital records or files. Desktop videoconferencing was the least tested mode because a majority of federal agencies reported that they did not have such capabilities.

Figure 5: Agencies Reported Testing Various IT and Telecommunications Capabilities

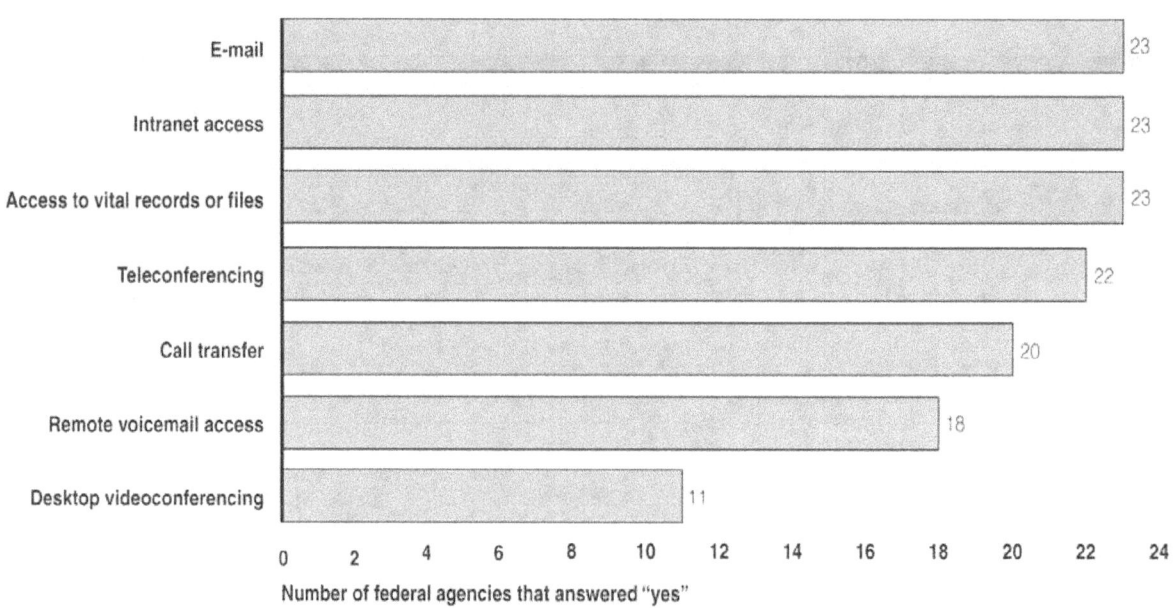

Source: GAO analysis of 2012 agency survey responses.

GAO-12-748 Influenza Pandemic

Many Agencies Reported Plans to Incorporate H1N1 Lessons Learned Into Influenza Pandemic Plans

We previously reported that it is important to recognize that agency influenza pandemic plans will continue to be revised and improved with additional time and information regarding influenza pandemic preparedness.[18] One recent event that prompted agencies to consider such revisions to their plans was the 2009 H1N1 influenza pandemic, which was the first human influenza pandemic in more than 4 decades.[19] Seventeen agencies reported in 2012 that they updated their influenza pandemic plan to include lessons learned from the pandemic. The Department of Energy (DOE), for example, reported that it had revised its plan to recommend that precautions and safeguards be based on the local prevalence of influenza at a specific DOE site rather than applying assumptions used for its headquarters location. HHS reported that following the first wave in the spring of 2009 and in anticipation of the second wave in the fall of 2009, HHS's Assistant Secretary for Administration convened a human capital task force to provide real-time solutions for key workforce related issues, including identification of departmental preparedness requirements and institutionalization of process and procedures. HHS also reported that after the 2009 H1N1 influenza pandemic, it had incorporated lessons learned that the task force identified as areas for improvement related to human capital into its draft influenza pandemic plan's human capital management and workforce protection annex. The areas where HHS has emphasized process improvement include the identification of mission critical employees that could work remotely and prompt communication of HHS's recommended actions for workforce protection and human capital plans to supervisors and employees.

Three agencies—the Department of Defense (DOD), Department of Veterans Affairs (VA), and National Science Foundation (NSF)—reported that they were planning to update their plans to include lessons learned from the 2009 H1N1 influenza pandemic during 2012 and 2013. In contrast, the Department of Agriculture (USDA), Department of Commerce (Commerce), SBA, and USAID, concluded that they did not have lessons learned from the 2009 H1N1 influenza pandemic

---

[18]GAO-09-404.

[19]In response to the global spread of the H1N1 influenza virus, the United Nations' World Health Organization declared the first human influenza pandemic in more than 4 decades on June 11, 2009. Prior to this declaration, H1N1 influenza had spread across the United States after first being detected in California in April 2009. The World Health Organization officially declared that the H1N1 pandemic was over in August 2010.

specifically related to workforce protection that warranted an update to their influenza pandemic plans.

Majority of Agencies Reported Various Influenza Pandemic Planning Activities at Component and Facility Levels

We reported in June 2009 that because the primary threat to continuity of operations during an influenza pandemic is the threat to employee health, agencies' plans to protect their workforce need to be operational at the facility level.[20] In addition, we reported that filtering influenza pandemic plans down to individual facilities and making them operational presented challenges for the agencies.[21]

A majority of agencies continued to report that they require pandemic plans at the component level, as shown in figure 6. Four agencies reported they did not require component level plans. The Department of Housing and Urban Development (HUD), OPM, and NSF reported in both 2009 and 2012 that they did not require their components to complete influenza pandemic plans. Although USAID reported in 2009 that it required its components to complete plans, the agency reported in 2012 that it uses a consolidated plan.

Figure 6: Majority of Agencies Reported Requiring Components to Complete Influenza Pandemic Plans

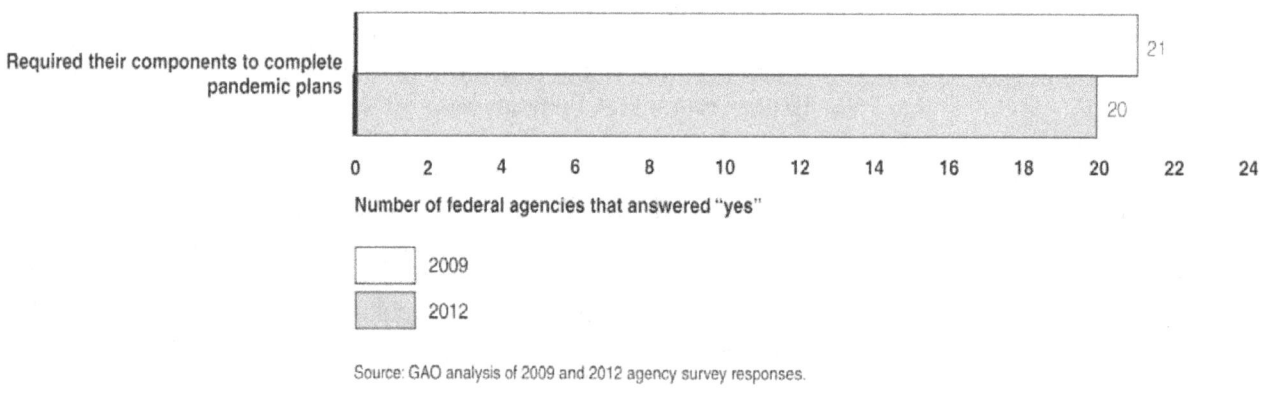

Source: GAO analysis of 2009 and 2012 agency survey responses.

---

[20]Facility refers to third-level entities subordinate to components such as service centers, inspection stations, and medical centers and clinics.

[21]GAO-09-404.

To better understand the extent to which influenza pandemic planning had filtered down to the component and facility levels, we included questions about these levels in our 2012 survey. For our 2012 survey, we selected one component from each of the 15 agencies who had provided examples of their key component-level mission essential functions that could not be performed remotely during an influenza pandemic in our 2009 survey, as shown in table 1.

Table 1: List of Agencies with Selected Components

Agency	Selected component
Department of Agriculture	Food Safety and Inspection Service
Department of Commerce	National Oceanic and Atmospheric Administration
Department of Energy	National Nuclear Security Administration
Department of Health and Human Services	National Institutes of Health
Department of Homeland Security	Customs and Border Protection
Department of Justice	Federal Bureau of Prisons
Department of Labor	Office of Workers' Compensation Programs
Department of State	Under Secretary for Management
Department of Transportation	Federal Aviation Administration
Department of the Treasury	U.S. Mint
Department of Veterans Affairs	National Cemetery Administration
Environmental Protection Agency	Region 10
National Aeronautics and Space Administration	Lyndon B. Johnson Space Center
Nuclear Regulatory Commission	Office of Nuclear Reactor Regulation
Social Security Administration	Office of the Deputy Commissioner, Operations

Source: GAO.

Figure 7 shows a high number of these agencies reported a broad level of activity in influenza pandemic planning for their selected components. Fourteen agencies reported that they have completed influenza pandemic plans that address how federal workers would be protected in the event of an influenza pandemic for their selected component and VA reported that its selected component, National Cemetery Administration, is covered under its departmental influenza pandemic plan and consequently does not need a separate component plan.

Figure 7: Selected Components' Influenza Pandemic Planning Efforts

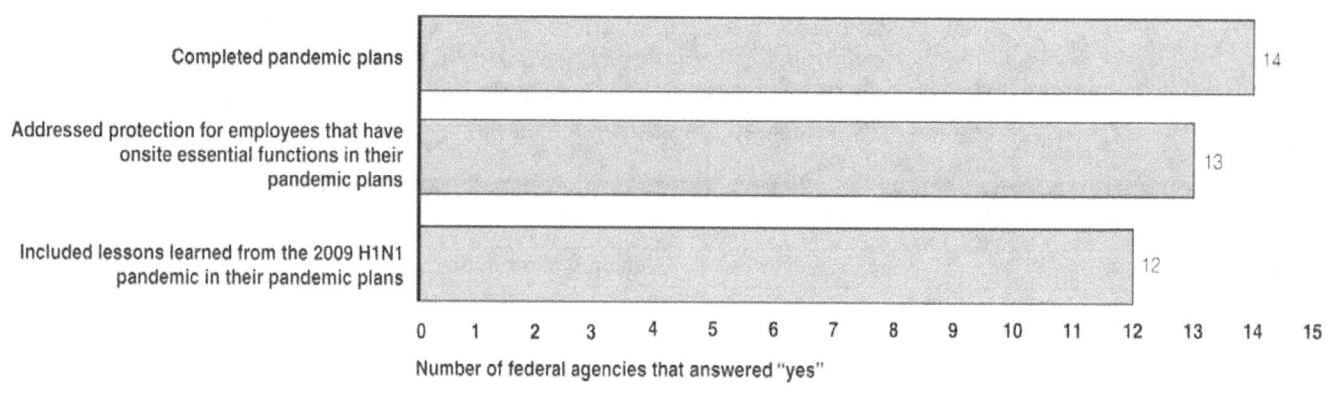

Number of federal agencies that answered "yes"

Source: GAO analysis of 2012 agency survey responses.

Of the 14 agencies with selected components that have plans, all but one reported they have addressed how employees who have onsite mission essential functions would be protected in the event of an influenza pandemic. The remaining agency, the Nuclear Regulatory Commission (NRC), reported that this was not applicable for its selected component, the Office of Nuclear Reactor Regulation (NRR), because NRR plans to perform all its mission essential functions remotely.

Further, 12 agencies with selected components reported they had incorporated lessons learned from the 2009 H1N1 influenza pandemic in their pandemic plans. Of the remaining two agencies with selected components that have plans, the Department of Transportation (DOT) reported that it has not yet incorporated lessons learned for its selected component, FAA, but is planning to incorporate them by the fall of 2012. In addition, Commerce reported that it does not plan on updating the National Oceanic and Atmospheric Administration's (NOAA) influenza pandemic plan to include lessons learned from the 2009 H1N1 influenza pandemic because there were no lessons specifically related to workforce protection that warranted a change. However, Commerce reported that NOAA will be reviewing its pandemic plan in late 2012.

The 14 agencies with selected components that have plans reported that all of the components included five of eight social distancing strategies to help reduce the risk of exposure for their employees, as shown in figure 8. As we mentioned earlier, avoiding crowded settings is one of the best ways to prevent infection during an influenza pandemic. However, not all of these actions may be applicable to all workplace settings.

Figure 8: Agencies Reported Using Various Social Distancing Strategies to Avoid Situations that Increase Workers' Risk of Exposure for Selected Components

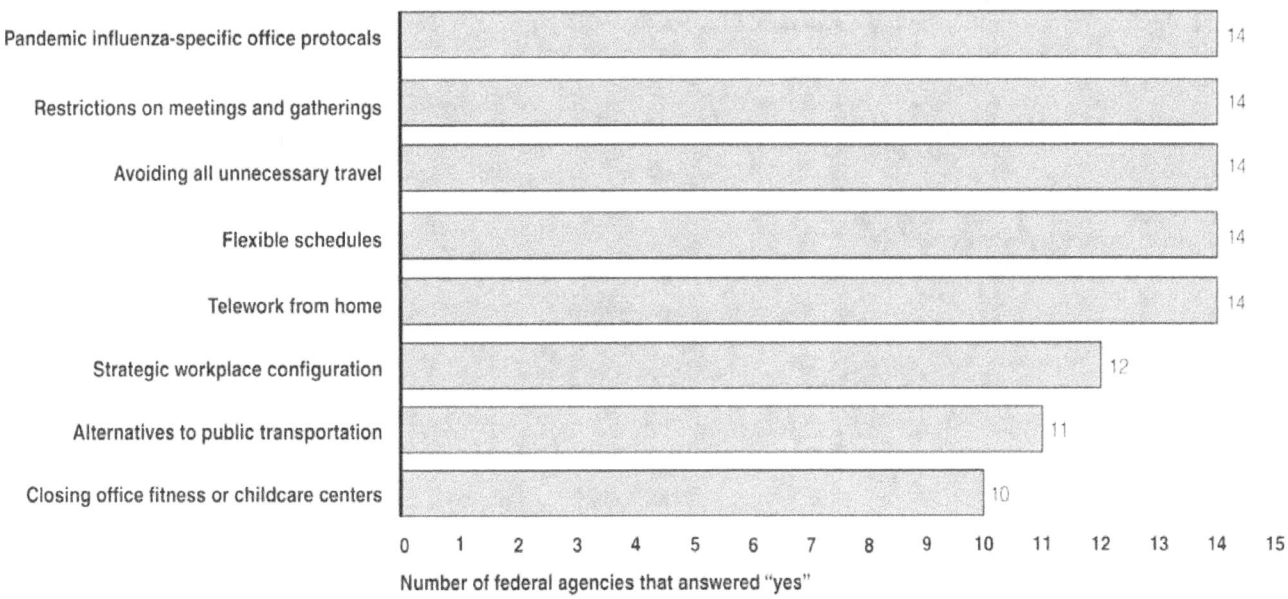

Number of federal agencies that answered "yes"

Source: GAO analysis of 2012 agency survey responses.

Figure 9 shows agency responses to our 2012 survey regarding influenza pandemic plans at the facility level.[22] Eight of the 15 agencies that have selected components have also required their facilities to complete influenza pandemic plans. The remaining seven agencies—Department of the Treasury (Treasury), HHS, Labor, National Aeronautics and Space Administration (NASA), NRC, Social Security Administration (SSA), and USDA—reported that they have not required facility-level plans for the components we had selected for a variety of reasons. For example, HHS, Labor, and Treasury reported they did not require their selected component's facilities to complete separate influenza pandemic plans

---

[22]Agencies reported a wide range of facilities for their selected component, including airport and seaport terminals, land border ports of entry, overseas U.S. embassies and consulates, and national cemeteries.

because they are covered under the component's plan, while NASA and NRC reported that it was not applicable because they have no facilities for the components we had selected. For example, NRC reported that NRR does not have facilities because it is located inside the main NRC headquarters complex.

Figure 9: Selected Components' Facility-Level Influenza Pandemic Plans

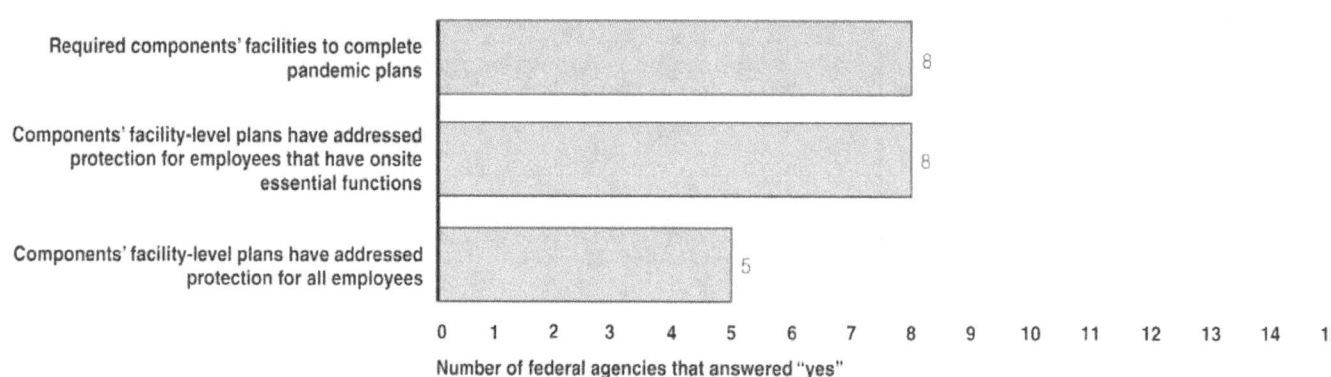

Number of federal agencies that answered "yes"

Source: GAO analysis of 2012 agency survey responses.

All of the eight agencies requiring components' facilities plans reported that these plans addressed how employees with onsite mission essential functions would be protected during an influenza pandemic. In addition, five of these eight agencies—DOE, Department of Justice, DOT, Environmental Protection Agency (EPA), and Department of State (State)—reported that all of their selected components' facilities plans addressed how employees would be protected in the event of an influenza pandemic. Of the remaining three, DHS reported that half or more of Customs and Border Protection's facilities addressed worker protection in their plans and Commerce and VA reported that some, but less than half, of their selected components' facilities have done so.

The use of various social distancing strategies reported in facilities' pandemic plans is highlighted in figure 10. As the figure shows, all eight of the agencies whose components' facilities were required to complete influenza pandemic plans also reported that their facility-level plans included social distancing strategies, such as implementing pandemic influenza-specific office protocols, restricting meetings and gatherings, and avoiding all unnecessary travel.

GAO-12-748 Influenza Pandemic

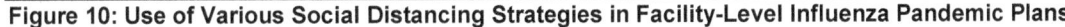

Figure 10: Use of Various Social Distancing Strategies in Facility-Level Influenza Pandemic Plans

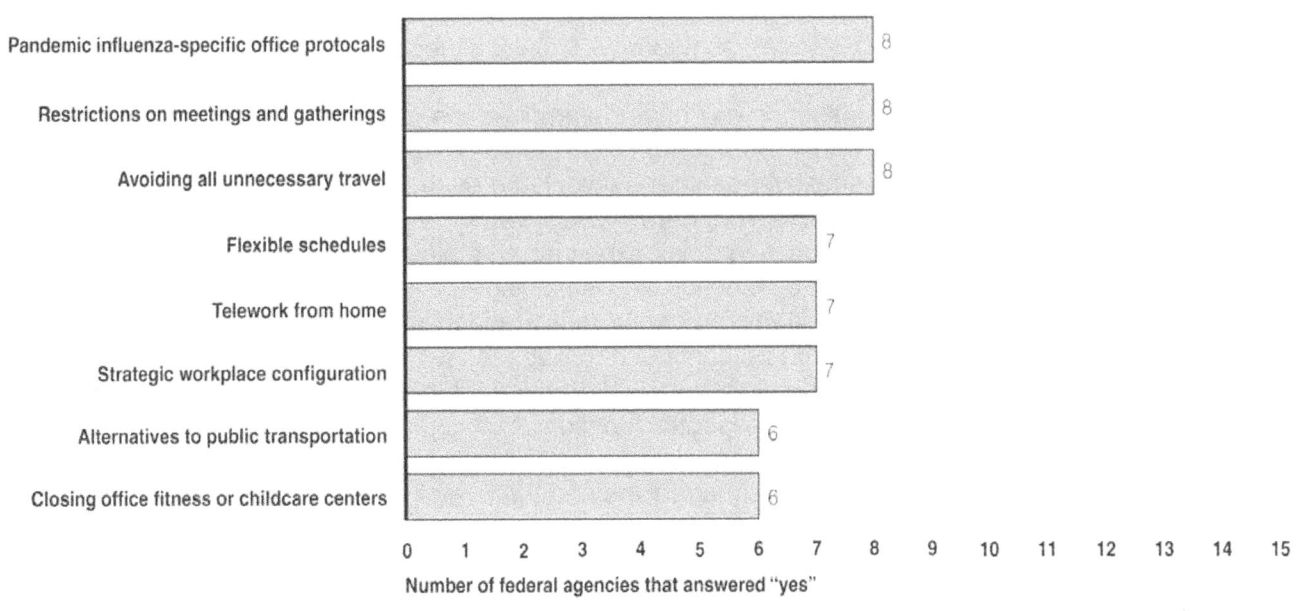

Number of federal agencies that answered "yes"

Source: GAO analysis of 2012 agency survey responses.

Many Agencies Reported Identification of Onsite Mission Essential Functions but Less than Half Reported Determining and Notifying Employees Tasked with Such Functions

Employees who must work onsite during an influenza pandemic will face varying levels of exposure risk. The level of risk depends, in part, on whether or not they will be in close proximity to people potentially infected with the influenza pandemic virus. OSHA has given guidance on steps employers can take to reduce the risk of exposure to influenza pandemic in their workplace.[23] For example, an agency could make changes to the work environment to reduce workplace hazards, such as installing sneeze guards between customers and employees to provide a barrier to transmission of the influenza virus. Additionally, an agency could provide personal protective equipment, such as surgical masks and N-95 respirators, to employees which, if used correctly, can help prevent some exposures. The steps that agencies could take to plan for appropriate employee protections include determining the number of employees they

---

[23]OSHA, *Guidance on Preparing Workplaces for an Influenza Pandemic.*

may need to protect, notifying those employees that may be expected to work, and classifying jobs by exposure risk level.

However, as figure 11 shows, although many of the agencies have identified mission essential functions that cannot be performed remotely, less than half have determined the number of employees that are tasked with performing onsite mission essential functions and notified the employees that they would be expected to work onsite during an influenza pandemic. Labor reported using a methodology of determining occupational risk exposure and telework designations by position rather than by function and is not represented in figure11. Through this methodology, Labor does not identify mission essential functions that cannot be continued through telework in the event of an influenza pandemic but does determine the number of its employees who perform mission essential functions that cannot be continued through telework. Labor reports that the notification of employees is a responsibility of its component agencies and the extent to which this has been completed is not known at the department level.

Figure 11: Agencies Reported Identification of Onsite Mission Essential Functions and Determination and Notification of Employees Tasked With Such Functions

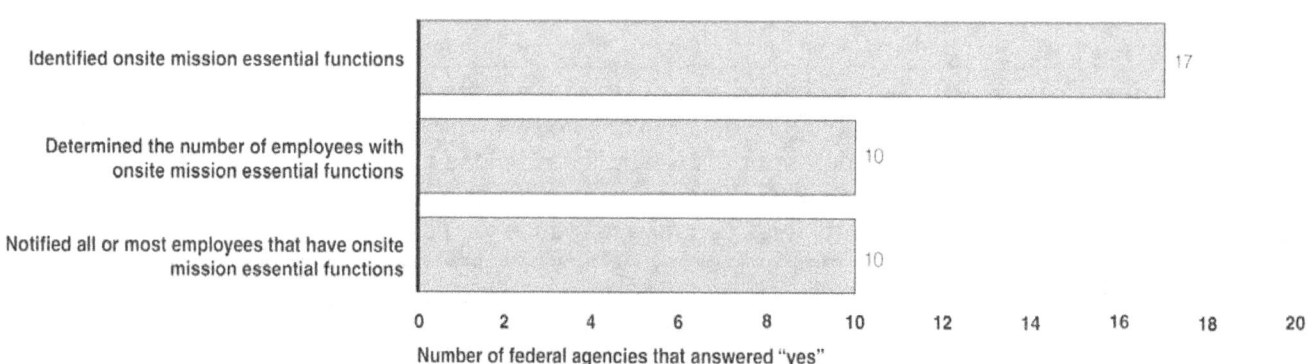

Source: GAO analysis of 2012 agency survey responses.

Note: This figure includes only 20 of 24 agencies. Of the remaining four agencies, Education, GSA, and SBA reported they could perform all of their mission essential functions remotely and Labor reported that it determines occupational risk exposure and telework designations by position rather than by mission essential function.

Seventeen agencies reported that they have identified which mission essential functions could not be performed remotely while EPA, HUD, and USAID reported that they were still in the process of determining them.

Ten of 17 agencies have determined the number of employees that would perform mission essential functions in the event of an influenza pandemic. The remaining seven agencies that have identified onsite mission essential functions reported that they have not yet determined the number of employees that must perform such functions in the event of an influenza pandemic. For example, SSA reported that it has not determined which jobs could be performed remotely because the agency's telework policy has not been ratified in its labor contract.

Of the 10 agencies that have determined the number of employees that cannot work remotely, all of them reported that they had also notified all or most of their employees who may be expected to continue operations during an influenza pandemic, an increase of 1 agency over 2009.

As we reported in June 2009, agencies should prepare employees for the risks of performing onsite mission essential functions.[24] A key step in making these determinations is to classify jobs by exposure risk level for mission essential functions that cannot be performed remotely. As figure 12 shows, of the 21 agencies reporting jobs associated with mission essential functions that cannot be performed remotely, although 9 agencies reported that they have classified all or most of their jobs by exposure risk level, 8 agencies reported having classified few or none. As noted earlier, Education, GSA, and SBA reported that all of their mission essential functions could be performed remotely.

---

[24]GAO-09-404.

Figure 12: Agencies Reported Uneven Status in Classifying Jobs by Exposure Risk Level for Onsite Mission Essential Functions

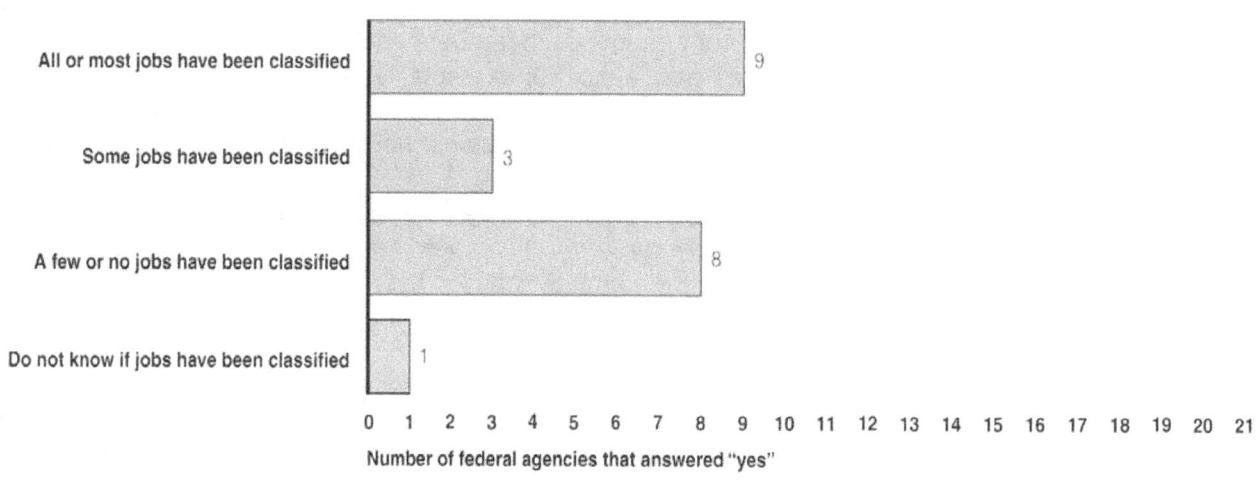

Source: GAO analysis of 2012 agency survey responses.

Note: This table does not include all 24 agencies because three of them reported they could perform all of their mission essential functions remotely.

Figure 13 shows that many agencies reported to have classified jobs that have onsite mission essential functions by exposure risk level for their selected component. Nine of the 14 agencies that have a selected component with onsite mission essential functions reported that they have classified all or most of their jobs by exposure risk level and only two agencies have classified a few or none. However, when compared to figure 12, agencies reported classifying jobs at the component level with onsite mission essential functions by exposure risk level to a greater degree than at the agency level.

Figure 13: Many Agencies Reported Classifying Jobs by Exposure Risk Level for Selected Component's Onsite Mission Essential Functions

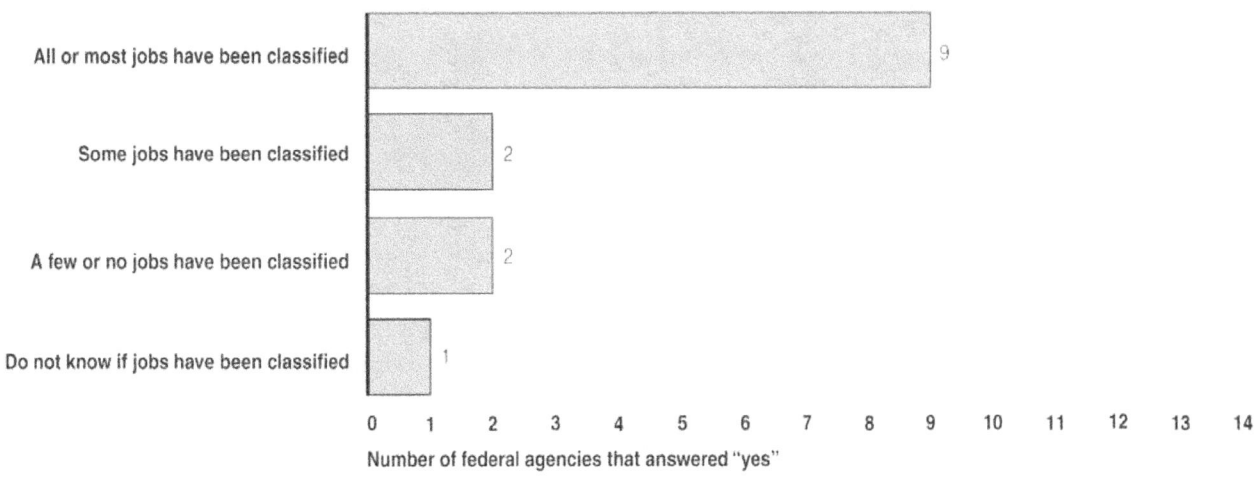

Number of federal agencies that answered "yes"

Source: GAO analysis of 2012 agency survey responses.

Note: This table does not include all 15 agencies with selected components because NRC reported that all of NRR's jobs could be performed remotely.

Twelve agencies and 11 selected components that completed or nearly completed the exposure risk classification also reported that they have specified the appropriate protection measures and could implement them, if instructed, to either a great extent or to some extent for those employees that cannot work remotely during an influenza pandemic.

Agencies Highlighted Various Challenges in Planning for an Influenza Pandemic

With the exception of DOD and Labor, 22 agencies identified various challenges in our 2012 survey that they faced in planning how to protect their workforce during an influenza pandemic. The top three challenges agencies most frequently cited, as shown in figure 14, were related to (1) medical countermeasures, such as antivirals and vaccines;[25] (2) information sharing; and (3) implementing various social distancing strategies.

---

[25]Medical countermeasures for use during an influenza pandemic may include vaccines, antiviral drugs, personal respirators, and influenza diagnostic tests. Vaccine, considered the first line of defense against influenza, is used to stimulate the production of an immune system response to protect the body from disease. Antiviral drugs are medications that can prevent or reduce the severity of a viral infection, such as influenza.

Figure 14: Most Frequently Reported Challenges in Planning for Federal Worker Protection for an Influenza Pandemic

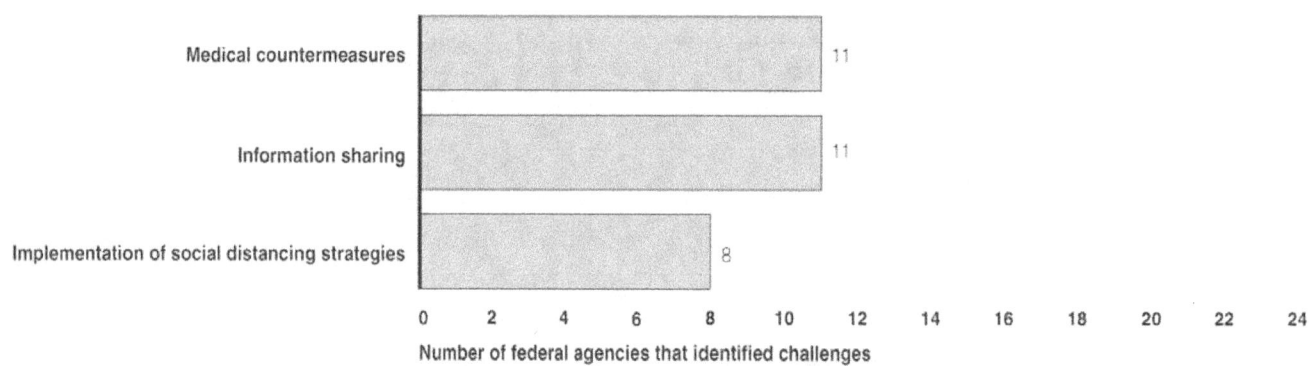

Number of federal agencies that identified challenges

Source: GAO analysis of 2012 agency survey responses.

Note: Two of the 24 agencies did not identify any challenges.

Almost half of the agencies, or 11, reported that understanding what actions they should take to procure, prioritize, and distribute vaccines and antivirals for their employees was a challenge. Specifically, some of these challenges included the lack of guidance related to policies and procedures for allocating and distributing vaccines and antivirals for their employees and how they should plan for nonfederal employees. For example, State reported that it had faced challenges because vaccines were not readily available during the 2009 H1N1 influenza pandemic for the approximately 50,000 employees and accompanying family members who work in embassies and consulates overseas. During the 2009 H1N1 influenza pandemic, State received a rationed shipment of vaccines for 2 percent of its workforce, which encompassed both domestic-based and international-based employees. The initial shipments were sent to State offices in Baghdad and Kabul; other diplomatic posts had to wait for later shipments. As we had reported in June 2011 on lessons learned from the 2009 H1N1 influenza pandemic, the H1N1 vaccine was not widely available when expected or when demand was highest in October 2009. By the time the H1N1 vaccine was widely available in late December 2009, the peak of H1N1 influenza activity had passed and many individuals were no longer as interested in getting vaccinated.[26] Further, DOT reported that there is a need for governmentwide guidance or

---

[26]GAO, *Influenza Pandemic: Lessons from the H1N1 Pandemic Should Be Incorporated into Future Planning*, GAO-11-632 (Washington, D.C.: June 27, 2011).

authority clarifying what federal agencies can legally do to protect onsite contractors who work closely with federal employees.

Unlike the allocation and distribution of seasonal influenza vaccines, the allocation and distribution of influenza pandemic vaccines are managed by the federal government. For example, during the 2009 H1N1 pandemic, the federal government determined that HHS would manage the allotment of the H1N1 vaccine. However, the federal agencies each make a decision whether or not to procure antivirals for their employees. Nevertheless, agencies still reported challenges. HHS reported that it issues nationwide guidance on the use of antivirals which informs the plans of employers who have chosen to stockpile these drugs, including federal agencies. However, HHS noted that it is an agency decision whether to purchase and distribute antivirals. HHS officials also acknowledged the lack of an approved process for internal HHS distribution of antivirals for its employees as a challenge, but noted they are evaluating lessons learned from the 2009 H1N1 influenza pandemic regarding this issue and will incorporate them into future influenza pandemic planning. Further, DOT reported that it had not planned for procuring antiviral medications for prophylaxis[27] because there is no requirement or reimbursement for federal agencies to do so; and SBA reported that stockpiling antivirals and prioritizing distribution of antivirals for its workforce, including who and when, were challenges.

Tied with medical countermeasures, 11 agencies cited challenges related to information sharing among federal agencies and also with their employees. For example, DOT and USDA reported they had not obtained post-H1N1 information regarding governmentwide lessons learned or best practices related to workforce protection issues that could be incorporated into their pandemic plans to help plan for future influenza pandemics. According to DHS's NRF, federal agencies should incorporate lessons learned from real-life incidents, such as an influenza pandemic, to make improvements in further strengthening their capability to respond to future emergencies.[28] The NRF specifies that evaluation

---

[27]Prophylactic use of medications is providing the medicine before an individual is diagnosed to help prevent or reduce the severity of a virus.

[28]Issued by DHS in January 2008, the NRF is the doctrine that guides how federal, state, local, and tribal governments, along with nongovernmental and private sector entities, will collectively respond to and recover from all-hazards, including catastrophic disasters such as Hurricane Katrina.

and continual process improvement are cornerstones of effective preparedness. We had previously recommended in June 2011 that the HSC should work with HHS, DHS, and other federal agencies to incorporate lessons learned from the 2009 H1N1 pandemic in addition to the lessons we identified, which included sharing relevant findings of agencies' after-action reports with key stakeholders, in planning for future pandemics.[29]

As noted earlier, agencies reported that there were challenges with communicating pandemic-related information to their employees. USDA, for example, reported that it was challenging to provide recurring pandemic-related information to ensure new employees were cognizant of its pandemic plans and guidance. In addition, HUD reported that providing real-time information to its employees could be a challenge, based on its experience with the 2009 H1N1 influenza pandemic. Further, HHS reported that it recognized that during the 2009 H1N1 influenza pandemic, its internal communication plans for workplace protection and human capital planning were delayed or inadequate. To address this shortfall, HHS's Centers for Disease Control and Prevention (CDC) and OPM published a communications toolkit during the 2009 H1N1 influenza pandemic in October 2009 for the federal workforce that included communications resources and guidance for federal employees and supervisors to use.[30] Our internal control standards for the federal government establish the need for relevant, reliable, and timely communications. According to these standards, effective communications should occur with information flowing down, across, and up the organization as well as with external stakeholders that may have a significant impact in meeting agency objectives.[31] Information sharing prior to and during an emergency, such as an influenza pandemic, is important to ensure the continuity of agencies' operations and mission essential functions.

Eight agencies reported that implementing various social distancing strategies, such as telework, workspace configuration, and IT capabilities,

---

[29]GAO-11-632.

[30]HHS, CDC, and OPM, *Preparing for the Flu: A Communications Toolkit for the Federal Workforce* (Oct. 1, 2009).

[31]GAO, *Standards for Internal Control in the Federal Government*, GAO/AIMD-00-21.3.1 (Washington, D.C.: November 1999).

was a challenge. Although we pointed out earlier that all 24 agencies reported that they planned to use telework as a means to protect their employees in the event of an influenza pandemic, several agencies reported that it may be a challenge to implement the measure. NASA, for instance, reported that because of the high level of commitment of its employees to assure mission success, educating and encouraging its workforce to use various social distancing recommendations, such as teleworking from home, canceling meetings, and not reporting to work when sick, was a challenge. In addition, NSF reported that it did not know whether all of its employees had internet capabilities in their homes to carry out work tasks remotely, while SBA reported that it was challenging to encourage all staff to become telework-enabled—such as having the appropriate capabilities at home to be able to work remotely. With respect to workspace configuration, DHS reported the difficulty of reconfiguring workspace to protect employees who must perform classified work in a sensitive compartmented information facility. Such facilities present similar social distancing challenges for air traffic controllers who work in close capacity in air route traffic control centers, which we will discuss next.

Pandemic Plans to Protect Air Traffic Controllers Have Progressed, but Social Distancing Remains an Intractable Challenge

We reported in 2009 that FAA pandemic plans to protect air traffic controllers were not ready for implementation and also highlighted various challenges in protecting air traffic controllers who had to perform onsite mission essential functions during an influenza pandemic. We followed up with FAA officials on the extent of their progress on four specific issues.

First, since our 2009 report, FAA has ensured that its facilities developed plans to protect air traffic controllers during an influenza pandemic. In 2009, we reported that the Air Traffic Organization (ATO), FAA's line of business responsible for air traffic controllers' services, had not directed facilities, such as its air route traffic control centers, to develop pandemic-specific plans. ATO directed its facilities 3 months after our report was issued to develop contingency staffing plans to mitigate the probable impact of an influenza pandemic and also instructed its facilities on immediate preparedness steps at the facility level.[32] For example, ATO

---

[32]The memorandum to ATO Senior Leadership from the Senior Vice President, Operations, on the subject of Immediate Preparedness Steps at the Facility and Office Level to Counter the Threat of Pandemic Influenza, Including the 2009 H1N1 Influenza Virus was issued on September 23, 2009.

facility managers were instructed to identify employees who were eligible and willing to telework, ensure that the appropriate employees complete the FAA telework program, and identify the minimum cadre of employees, by position, who would need to telework during an influenza pandemic outbreak to sustain mission essential services.

Second, FAA augmented its agencywide pandemic plan with a workplace protection policy. In 2010, FAA updated ATO's draft pandemic plan with detailed protective measures for its workforce, including air traffic controllers.[33] For example, FAA added information to the plan about sanitizers that are safe to use on air traffic control equipment. At the time of our report in 2009, FAA had not yet certified a sanitizer to be used to sanitize the equipment. It was important for FAA to certify a sanitizer because many sanitizers are caustic and could corrode sensitive equipment necessary for flight safety. ATO's plan now states employees should regularly cleanse shared equipment using certified disinfectant or cleaning agents. Additional measures call for employees to take a pandemic awareness course, cover coughs, and wash their hands frequently, which are consistent with CDC's guidance. FAA reported the plan has been distributed as guidance to managers and supervisors and remains in draft status as it is a "living document."

Third, FAA has addressed issues related to medication. At the time of our report in 2009, the Office of Aerospace Medicine had not finalized its policy on the preventative use of the flu medication Tamiflu by on-duty controllers. FAA regulations on medication for air traffic controllers are strict because certain medications may impair air traffic controllers' performance. The Office of Aerospace Medicine revised and finalized its policy in 2009 regarding the use of Tamiflu for preventative use by on-duty controllers.[34] FAA will allow air traffic controllers to continue to work if they have been prescribed antiviral medications by either a public health authority or their personal physicians, if no side effects from the medications are evident, and if they are operating normally on the job.

---

[33]FAA, *Air Traffic Organization: Implementation Plan for Sustaining Essential Government Services During an Influenza Pandemic* (Jan. 5, 2010).

[34]FAA, *Use of Anti-Influenza Medication by FAA Employees Performing Safety-Related Duties* (Oct. 8, 2009).

Finally, FAA was not able to resolve social distancing challenges. CDC recommends maintaining 6 feet of separation during an influenza pandemic, but this is not possible for air traffic controllers because they work in close quarters. According to FAA officials, they considered having air traffic controllers use personal protective equipment, but concluded that N-95 respirators or surgical masks impede the clear verbal communications necessary to maintain aviation safety. At the time of our report in 2009, FAA had just received the results of a feasibility study for the use of a powered air purifying respirator. The study findings suggested that if FAA used the technology, it would need to address many potential problems including noise, visibility, and comfort. At this time, FAA officials state they have not identified a technical solution to equip controllers with a practical protective piece of equipment that will mitigate the risk of working in close quarters while supporting adequate communications necessary for safety. The FAA official responsible for ATO's pandemic planning stated social distancing challenges appear intractable with the current technology, although FAA will continue to seek opportunities to mitigate potential exposure to influenza. For the present, this includes being vigilant in implementing hygiene measures in their workspaces and exploring other mitigation controls such as technological advances that reduce transmissibility.

Agencies' Plans and Progress to Protect Federal Workers during an Influenza Pandemic Receive Limited Oversight

Federal Continuity Directive 1 requires federal executive agency heads to evaluate program readiness to ensure the adequacy and capability of continuity plans and programs. In addition, the agency head must submit an annual report to the National Continuity Coordinator (NCC) to certify the agency has this capability. As previously discussed, all agencies reported having completed influenza pandemic agency plans.

Under the HSC's Implementation Plan, DHS was charged with, among other things, monitoring and reporting to the President on the readiness of departments and agencies to continue their operations while protecting their workers during an influenza pandemic. However, DHS officials said the HSC informed them in late 2006 or early 2007 that they were not required to report on these responsibilities. Rather, the HSC requested that agencies certify to the council that their plans addressed the applicable elements of a pandemic checklist in 2006 and again in 2008. However, according to two agencies' officials, the HSC has not asked agencies to certify their plans since then. As we reported in 2011, the National Security Staff (NSS), who supports the HSC, is coordinating a larger effort to transition national preparedness from a dependence on fixed plans for specific threats to an approach based on a variety of hazards, or an all-hazards approach in accordance with Presidential Policy Directive 8.[35,36,37] We submitted a request for information and asked to meet with the relevant NSS subject matter experts regarding oversight of agencies' preparedness to protect workers during a pandemic. An NSS official advised that the NSS would not be able to provide responsive information because these issues are currently being addressed through the Presidential Policy Directive 1 process.[38] Officials at two agencies we spoke with informed us that the NSS has reconvened the Pandemic Preparedness Sub-Interagency Policy Coordination Committee to primarily address domestic pandemic preparedness efforts, with a focus on coordination between departments and agencies. In the absence of any information from the HSC, it is not possible to determine what, if anything, it is doing to oversee federal agency pandemic planning. Regarding the 2009 recommendation we made to the HSC, DHS officials told us that the HSC has not requested the Secretary of Homeland Security to monitor and report to the President on the readiness of agencies to continue their operations while protecting their employees in the event of a pandemic.

As we did in 2009, we interviewed four agencies to which the Implementation Plan assigns responsibilities related to pandemic

---

[35]GAO-11-632.

[36]On May 26, 2009, the President established the NSS, under the direction of the National Security Advisor, to integrate White House staff supporting national security and homeland security. The President stated that the NSS would support the HSC, and that the HSC would be maintained as the principal venue for interagency deliberations on issues that affect the security of the homeland, such as pandemic influenza. See *Statement by the President on the White House Organization for Homeland Security and Terrorism*, accessed July 17, 2012, http://www.whitehouse.gov/the_press_office/Statement-by-the-President-on-the-White-House-Organization-for-Homeland-Security-and-Counterterrorism.

[37]Issued in March 30, 2011 by the President, the Presidential Policy Directive 8 documents that the Secretary of Homeland Security is responsible for coordinating the domestic all-hazards preparedness efforts of all executive departments and agencies and for developing the national preparedness goal.

[38]Issued in February 2009 by the President, the Presidential Policy Directive 1 documents the organization of the National Security Council (NSC), which is the principal forum for consideration of national security policy issues requiring presidential determination. The NSC is the President's principal means for coordinating executive departments and agencies in the development and implementation of national security policy. Management of development and implementation of national security policies by multiple agencies of the U.S. government shall be accomplished by the NSC Interagency Policy Committees.

preparedness. The four agencies we selected are responsible for providing guidance, policy, or influenza pandemic-related expertise to other agencies. Each of these agencies is responsible for providing influenza pandemic continuity of operations (COOP) guidance, which includes elements such as COOP planning, personnel protection, or workplace options for federal departments and agencies.

- Labor's OSHA is responsible for promoting the safety and health of workers, including communication of information related to an influenza pandemic to workers and employers.[39]
- HHS is responsible for the overall coordination of the public health and medical emergency response during an influenza pandemic. HHS communicates information related to an influenza pandemic, ensures provision of essential human services, implements measures to limit the spread of influenza, provides recommendations related to the use, distribution, and allocation of influenza countermeasures, and to the provision of care in mass casualty settings.[40]
- OPM, in coordination with DHS, HHS, DOD, and Labor, provides guidance to federal departments and agencies on human capital management[41] and COOP planning criteria related to an influenza pandemic.
- DHS coordinates the overall domestic federal response during an influenza pandemic, including implementing policies that facilitate compliance with recommended social distancing measures, developing a common operating picture for all federal agencies, and ensuring the integrity of the nation's infrastructure.

---

[39]OSHA issued *Guidance on Preparing Workplaces for an Influenza Pandemic* in 2007 for employers and employees, to help identify risk levels in workplace settings and appropriate control measures that include good hygiene, cough etiquette, social distancing, the use of personal protective equipment and staying home from work when ill.

[40]HHS's *H1N1 Compendium,* designed to be utilized by healthcare providers and practitioners, provides guidance on the interventions for H1N1 in the emergency and "first care" provider infrastructure throughout the United States. The compendium provides specific recommendations, consultation, and guidance on various matters, including: hospital best practices, hospital intervention trigger points for pandemic responses, H1N1 intervention guidance, screening guidelines, and equipment/supply recommendations. For example, CDC provides additional guidance by audience and updates based on lessons learned.

[41]The U.S. government website, accessed July 17, 2012, http://www.flu.gov contains information for federal employees, human resources practitioners, and managers on human capital policies in effect during an influenza pandemic such as flexible work arrangements, health benefits, and leave and pay flexibilities.

GAO-12-748 Influenza Pandemic

DHS does not conduct oversight of agencies' plans as originally envisioned in the Implementation Plan, and DHS officials responsible for coordinating organizational roles and responsibilities related to these responsibilities confirmed that DHS does not specifically provide oversight of agencies' influenza pandemic plans. But these officials told us that DHS is the federal lead agency for coordinating overall continuity operations.[42] In this capacity, DHS coordinates the assessment of agencies' continuity activities and programs. The DHS Secretary provides biennial assessments of department and agency continuity capabilities and reports the results to the President, through the NCC, and to agency heads as required by Federal Continuity Directive 1.[43]

FEMA officials responsible for the national continuity program noted that while agencies are responsible for their preparedness, and FEMA does not assess the efficacy of overall agency pandemic preparedness, FEMA's biennial assessment process does assess whether agencies' continuity plans address some of the unique considerations of an influenza pandemic. FEMA collects agency information for the assessment through continuity exercises and the *Continuity Evaluation Tool* (evaluation tool), a comprehensive survey covering 14 elements of continuity programs, plans, and procedures for all-hazards, including a pandemic threat. In addition to reporting to the NCC, FEMA also compares the results of multiple biennial continuity assessments to identify government trends in overall continuity preparedness. The evaluation tool asks whether agencies' communications capabilities will allow them to continue operations for all types of emergencies, including influenza pandemics. The evaluation tool also asks if agencies have given full consideration to social distancing strategies, such as telework. Because the evaluation tool which FEMA uses to evaluate agencies' continuity plans is based on an all-hazards approach, it does not include the planning elements identified in the Key Elements checklist that agencies specifically use for pandemic planning. Consequently, the evaluation tool, for example, does not include pandemic preparedness-related questions such as whether federal workers' influenza pandemic

---

[42]Within DHS, FEMA is responsible for preparing and implementing the plans and programs of the federal government for the continuity of operations pursuant to 6 U.S.C. § 314.

[43]DHS released the Federal Continuity Directive 1 in February 2008 to provide direction for the development of continuity plans and programs for the federal executive branch.

risk assessments are regularly updated and whether agencies have planned to provide protective measures to mitigate exposure risks.

Conclusions

Our follow-up survey of the 24 CFO Act agencies showed that significant progress has been made in many areas since we last reported on this issue in 2009. In particular, almost all or most of the agencies, selected components, and their facilities have completed pandemic plans that address how they would protect employees that were associated with mission essential functions that could not be performed remotely. In addition, almost half of the agencies reported to have determined the number of employees that would have to perform mission essential functions and also notified the employees that they were expected to continue these operations during an influenza pandemic. However, the agencies also reported uneven status in some key areas suggesting some oversight targeted to bring attention to these areas is needed. For example, only nine agencies reported that they have classified all or most jobs for onsite mission essential functions by exposure risk level. Given the continued threat of an influenza pandemic, it is important that agencies have operational pandemic plans that identify appropriate workforce strategies to protect employees while ensuring mission essential functions continue. Adequate oversight could help in ensuring that, by classifying jobs by exposure risk level, agencies have appropriate measures in place to protect those employees who must carry out mission essential functions that cannot be performed remotely during an influenza pandemic.

Agencies reported several challenges in planning for federal worker protection in the event of an influenza pandemic. Sharing of information among agencies is related to some of these challenges. The Pandemic Preparedness Sub-Interagency Policy Coordination Committee meetings led by the NSS may provide a venue and opportunity to identify agencies' needs and improve coordination to address gaps the agencies perceive in guidance and pandemic-related information needs.

FAA has made progress in three of the four areas related to protecting air traffic controllers we highlighted as challenges in 2009. However, FAA has not yet found a viable way to address how onsite air traffic controllers, who work in close proximity to each other, could be separated during an influenza pandemic. Further, FAA has not yet identified personal protective equipment alternatives for use by air traffic controllers who must report to work during an influenza pandemic. These issues will continue to be challenges for which FAA may not be able to find viable solutions.

FEMA's biennial assessment of agencies' continuity capabilities does not consider agency responses to significant influenza pandemic-related questions regarding protection of federal workers. Such questions may include whether jobs have been classified by exposure risk level and whether appropriate protective measures have been identified and will be available as needed for their employees. While agencies have reported in 2012 they have made significant progress in planning for protecting workers during an influenza pandemic, additional oversight targeted to those areas in which reported progress is uneven could help focus attention on those areas. The existing biennial assessment process provides an opportunity to provide monitoring, evaluation and reporting on protecting federal workers during an influenza pandemic.

Recommendation For Executive Action

To provide additional oversight of agencies' progress in their preparedness to protect workers, help focus attention on areas of uneven progress reported in our survey, and build upon the efforts FEMA has underway, we recommend that the Secretary of Homeland Security direct the Administrator of FEMA to include in its biennial assessments of agencies' continuity capabilities consideration of agencies' progress in assessing exposure risk levels, identifying appropriate protective measures, and establishing operational plans to provide such protections.

Agency Comments

We provided the Secretary of Homeland Security with a draft of this report for review and comment. In written comments, the Director of the Departmental GAO-Office of the Inspector General Liaison Office concurred with the recommendation and stated that DHS is committed to ensuring COOP programs continue to focus on all-hazards, including pandemic planning, in an evolving environment. As part of this commitment, FEMA reviews its *Continuity Evaluation Tool* on a regular basis and will update it to provide specific attention to pandemic planning within the context of all-hazard planning, including assessing the risk of pandemic impacts to specific functions, identifying protective measures for employees performing those functions, and planning for providing protection, as appropriate. Technical comments were also provided, which we incorporated. DHS's comments are reprinted in appendix IV.

As agreed with your office, unless you publicly announce the contents of this report earlier, we plan no further distribution until 30 days from the report date. We are sending copies of this report to the Department of Homeland Security; relevant congressional committees; and other interested parties. The report also is available at no charge on the GAO website at http://www.gao.gov.

If you or your staff members have any questions about this report, please contact me at (202) 512-9110 or czerwinskis@gao.gov. Contact points for our Offices of Congressional Relations and Public Affairs may be found on the last page of this report. GAO staff who made major contributions to this report are listed in appendix V.

Stanley J. Czerwinski
Director, Strategic Issues

Appendix I: Chief Financial Officers Act Agencies

- Department of Agriculture
- Department of Commerce
- Department of Defense
- Department of Education
- Department of Energy
- Department of Health and Human Services
- Department of Homeland Security
- Department of Housing and Urban Development
- Department of the Interior
- Department of Justice
- Department of Labor
- Department of State
- Department of Transportation
- Department of the Treasury
- Department of Veterans Affairs
- Environmental Protection Agency
- General Services Administration
- National Aeronautics and Space Administration
- National Science Foundation
- Nuclear Regulatory Commission
- Office of Personnel Management
- Small Business Administration
- Social Security Administration
- U.S. Agency for International Development

Appendix II: List of Agencies and Selected Components

Agency	Selected component
Department of Agriculture	Food Safety and Inspection Service
Department of Commerce	National Oceanic and Atmospheric Administration
Department of Energy	National Nuclear Security Administration
Department of Health and Human Services	National Institutes of Health
Department of Homeland Security	Customs and Border Protection
Department of Justice	Federal Bureau of Prisons
Department of Labor	Office of Workers' Compensation Programs
Department of State	Under Secretary for Management
Department of Transportation	Federal Aviation Administration
Department of the Treasury	U.S. Mint
Department of Veterans Affairs	National Cemetery Administration
Environmental Protection Agency	Region 10
National Aeronautics and Space Administration	Lyndon B. Johnson Space Center
Nuclear Regulatory Commission	Office of the Nuclear Reactor Regulation
Social Security Administration	Office of the Deputy Commissioner, Operations

Source: GAO.

Appendix III: Objectives, Scope, and Methodology

The objectives of this report were to (1) determine what progress federal agencies report they have made since our 2009 report and identify challenges federal agencies report they face in protecting their workforce during an influenza pandemic, and (2) determine the extent to which oversight of agencies' progress was being conducted and how the oversight information is being used.

To address the first objective, we developed and administered a web-based survey of the 24 agencies covered by the Chief Financial Officers Act of 1990 (CFO Act) to determine to what extent they had made progress in their preparedness to protect their workforce for an influenza pandemic since our 2009 survey and to identify challenges they faced in planning for protection of their workers. We developed the survey questions based on guidelines for worker protection from the Homeland Security Council (HSC), Department of Health and Human Services (HHS), Federal Emergency Management Agency (FEMA), Occupational Safety and Health Administration (OSHA), and Office of Personnel Management (OPM), and we also used some of the survey questions we asked in 2009. The survey included questions related to (1) pandemic plans, (2) mission essential functions that could not be continued through telework during an influenza pandemic, (3) assessment of levels of exposure risk, (4) measures planned to protect workers who would not be able to work remotely, (5) social distancing strategies, (6) testing of information technology and telecommunications capabilities, (7) communication of human capital pandemic policies, (8) oversight of pandemic planning, and (9) challenges in planning for worker protection.

To better understand the extent to which influenza pandemic planning had filtered down to the component and facility levels, we also gathered data from these levels in our 2012 survey. In our 2009 survey, 15 of 24 agencies provided examples of some of the key component-level mission essential functions that could not be performed remotely during an influenza pandemic. Using those examples, we selected a component from each of these 15 agencies for our 2012 survey and surveyed the agencies to determine whether they had made plans at lower organizational levels to protect their employees whose onsite presence was necessary in order to carry out mission essential functions.

Prior to disseminating our web-based survey, we conducted a series of pretests from November 16 through November 21, 2011, with three agencies to further refine our questions, clarify any ambiguous portions of the survey, and identify potentially biased questions. Upon completion of the pretests and development of the final survey questions and format,

we sent an announcement of the upcoming survey to the 24 CFO Act
agencies on December 12, 2011. These agencies were notified that the
survey was available online on December 14, 2011. We sent reminder e-
mail messages to nonrespondents on January 3, 2012, and January 9,
2012. The survey was available online until January 13, 2012, and the
results were confirmed or updated through June 2012. All 24 CFO Act
agencies completed the survey for a response rate of 100 percent.

Furthermore, we reviewed the *National Strategy for Pandemic Influenza
Implementation Plan*, *National Response Framework*, our prior work
assessing influenza, and other relevant literature. We defined mission
essential functions based on the Department of Homeland Security's
(DHS) Federal Continuity Directive 1 as those functions that enable an
organization to provide vital services, exercise civil authority, maintain the
safety of the general public, and sustain the industrial and economic base
during disruption of normal operations. The scope of our work did not
include an independent evaluation of the effectiveness of the workforce
protection measures recommended by federal lead pandemic agencies.

In addition to the survey, we conducted follow-up work to determine
whether the Federal Aviation Administration had made progress in
addressing the unique challenges we highlighted in our 2009 report
regarding protection for air traffic controllers who must perform onsite
mission essential functions during an influenza pandemic. We reviewed
agency and component pandemic plans and conducted interviews with
agency officials.

To address the second objective, we analyzed documentation of
oversight activities and our prior work, and conducted interviews with
officials from DHS, HHS, FEMA, OPM, and OSHA, who were tasked with
providing guidance, policy, or influenza pandemic related expertise to
other federal agencies in planning for an influenza pandemic.

We conducted this performance audit from July 2011 through July 2012 in
accordance with generally accepted government auditing standards.
Those standards require that we plan and perform the audit to obtain
sufficient, appropriate evidence to provide a reasonable basis for our
findings and conclusions based on our audit objectives. We believe that
the evidence obtained provides a reasonable basis for our findings and
conclusions based on our audit objectives.

Appendix IV: Comments from the Department of Homeland Security

U.S. Department of Homeland Security
Washington, D.C. 20528

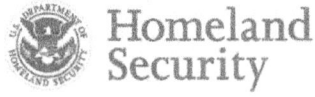

July 9, 2012

Stanley J. Czerwinski
Director, Strategic Issues
U.S. Government Accountability Office
441 G Street, NW
Washington, DC 20548

Re: Draft Report GAO-12-748, "INFLUENZA PANDEMIC: Agencies Report Progress
         in Plans to Protect Federal Workers but Oversight Could Be Improved"

Dear Mr. Czerwinski:

Thank you for the opportunity to review and comment on this draft report. The U.S. Department of
Homeland Security (DHS) appreciates the U.S. Government Accountability Office's (GAO's) work
in planning and conducting its review and issuing this report.

The Department is pleased to note GAO's positive recognition that federal agencies have made
significant progress since 2009 in planning to protect employees during an influenza pandemic.
This increase in planning by 23 of 24 agencies reviewed further assures a viable capability exists
for agencies to perform Mission Essential Functions as part of their Continuity of Operations
(COOP) programs when needed.

The draft report contained one recommendation with which the Department concurs.
Specifically, GAO recommended that the Secretary of Homeland Security:

Recommendation: Direct the Administrator of FEMA to include in its biennial assessments of
agencies' continuity capabilities consideration of agencies' progress in assessing exposure risk
levels, identifying appropriate protective measures, and establishing operational plans to provide
such protections.

Response: Concur. DHS is committed to ensuring COOP programs continue to focus on all
hazards, including pandemic planning, in an evolving environment. As part of this
commitment, the Federal Emergency Management Agency (FEMA) reviews its Continuity
Evaluation Tool (CET) on a regular basis. The CET is a critical tool for agencies to use when
conducting annual self-assessments of their COOP plans. In addition, the CET serves as the
guide for independent, external evaluation of the continuity capability of federal departments
and agencies as part of the biennial government-wide operations-based exercise, Eagle
Horizon.

FEMA will update the CET to provide specific attention to pandemic planning within the
context of all-hazard planning. The CET will address assessing the risk of pandemic impacts
to specific functions, identifying protective measures for employees performing those
functions, and planning for providing protection, as appropriate.

Again, thank you again for the opportunity to review and comment on this draft report.
Technical comments were previously provided under separate cover. Please feel free to
contact me if you have any questions. We look forward to working with you in the future.

Sincerely,

Jim H. Crumpacker
Director
Departmental GAO-OIG Liaison Office

2

Appendix V: GAO Contact and Staff Acknowledgments

GAO Contact	Stanley J. Czerwinski, (202) 512-9110 or czerwinskis@gao.gov
Staff Acknowledgments	In addition to the contact named above, William J. Doherty, Assistant Director; Maya Chakko; David Dornisch; Karin Fangman; Robert Gebhart; Stuart Kaufman; Ruben Montes de Oca; Patricia Norris; Susan Sato; and Andrew Stavisky made major contributions to this report. Ellen Grady and Judith Kordahl verified the information in the report.

Related GAO Products

Influenza Pandemic: Lessons from the H1N1 Pandemic Should Be Incorporated into Future Planning. GAO-11-632. Washington, D.C.: June 27, 2011.

Influenza Vaccine: Federal Investments in Alternative Technologies and Challenges to Development and Licensure. GAO-11-435. Washington, D.C.: June 27, 2011.

Disaster Response: Criteria for Developing and Validating Effective Response Plans. GAO-10-969T. Washington, D.C.: September 22, 2010.

Influenza Pandemic: Monitoring and Assessing the Status of the National Pandemic Implementation Plan Needs Improvement. GAO-10-73. Washington, D.C.: November 24, 2009.

Influenza Pandemic: Gaps in Pandemic Planning and Preparedness Need to Be Addressed. GAO-09-909T. Washington, D.C.: July 29, 2009.

Influenza Pandemic: Increased Agency Accountability Could Help Protect Federal Employees Serving the Public in the Event of a Pandemic. GAO-09-404. Washington, D.C.: June 12, 2009.

Influenza Pandemic: Continued Focus on the Nation's Planning and Preparedness Efforts Remains Essential. GAO-09-760T. Washington, D.C.: June 3, 2009.

Influenza Pandemic: Sustaining Focus on the Nation's Planning and Preparedness Efforts. GAO-09-334. Washington, D.C.: February 26, 2009.

Influenza Pandemic: HHS Needs to Continue Its Actions and Finalize Guidance for Pharmaceutical Interventions. GAO-08-671. Washington, D.C.: September 30, 2008.

Influenza Pandemic: Efforts Under Way to Address Constraints on Using Antivirals and Vaccines to Forestall a Pandemic. GAO-08-92. Washington, D.C.: December 21, 2007.

Influenza Vaccine: Issues Related to Production, Distribution, and Public Health Messages. GAO-08-27. Washington, D.C.: October 31, 2007.

Influenza Pandemic: Further Efforts Are Needed to Ensure Clearer Federal Leadership Roles and an Effective National Strategy. GAO-07-781. Washington, D.C.: August 14, 2007.

Influenza Pandemic: Efforts to Forestall Onset Are Under Way; Identifying Countries at Greatest Risk Entails Challenges. GAO-07-604. Washington, D.C.: June 20, 2007.

Influenza Pandemic: Applying Lessons Learned from the 2004–05 Influenza Vaccine Shortage. GAO-06-221T. Washington, D.C.: November 4, 2005.

Influenza Vaccine: Shortages in 2004–05 Season Underscore Need for Better Preparation. GAO-05-984. Washington, D.C.: September 30, 2005.

Influenza Pandemic: Challenges in Preparedness and Response. GAO-05-863T. Washington, D.C.: June 30, 2005.

Influenza Pandemic: Challenges Remain in Preparedness. GAO-05-760T. Washington, D.C.: May 26, 2005.

www.ingramcontent.com/pod-product-compliance
Lightning Source LLC
Chambersburg PA
CBHW080914290526
45795CB00007BA/2523